FART
OPEDIA

SUMMERSDALE PUBLISHERS LTD
46 WEST STREET
CHICHESTER
WEST SUSSEX
PO19 1RP
UK

WWW.SUMMERSDALE.COM

PRINTED AND BOUND IN THE CZECH REPUBLIC

ISBN: 978-1-84953-740-7

SUBSTANTIAL DISCOUNTS ON BULK QUANTITIES OF SUMMERSDALE BOOKS ARE AVAILABLE TO CORPORATIONS, PROFESSIONAL ASSOCIATIONS AND OTHER ORGANISATIONS. FOR DETAILS CONTACT NICKY DOUGLAS BY TELEPHONE: +44 (O) 1243 756902, FAX: +44 (O) 1243 786300 OR EMAIL: NICKY@SUMMERSDALE.COM.

FARTOPEDIA

EVERYTHING YOU DIDN'T NEED TO KNOW — AND MORE!

MARTIN FLEMING

summersdale

CONTENTS

INTRODUCTION

WE ALL DO IT, ALTHOUGH SOME OF US FART QUIETLY IN PRIVATE WHILE OTHERS TRUMP PROUDLY FOR ALL TO ENJOY – IN A BOARD MEETING, ON THE TRAIN OR IN A LIFT (MY PERSONAL FAVOURITE). FOR THE FIRST TIME, AFTER YEARS OF PAINSTAKING RESEARCH, FARTS HAVE BEEN DISTILLED AND EXPLAINED IN THE WORLD'S FIRST *FARTOPEDIA*. KEEP IT WITH YOU AT ALL TIMES SO THE NEXT TIME YOU HEAR OR SMELL A TRUMP YOU'LL BE ABLE TO IDENTIFY IT – YOU'LL WONDER HOW YOU EVER LIVED WITHOUT THIS FABULOUS TOME.

FART RATINGS

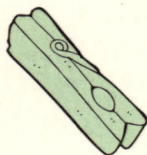

SMELLINESS RATING: FARTS THAT SCORE HIGHLY IN THIS RATING ARE BOUND TO MAKE YOUR EYES WATER. SOME FARTS ARE SO VILE YOU'D THINK THEY'D BE ACCOMPANIED BY A GREEN FOG INSTEAD OF JUST THE PUTRID STENCH THAT FILLS THE ROOM. A TRADITIONAL WAY OF ESCAPING THIS ELEMENT OF A FART IS A GOOD OLD-FASHIONED CLOTHES PEG ON THE NOSE, SO THE SMELL OF A FART IN THIS BOOK IS MEASURED IN PEGS.

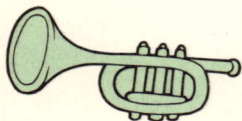

LOUDNESS RATING: FARTS THAT EXCEL HERE WILL CERTAINLY NOT GO QUIETLY, ANNOUNCING THEIR ARRIVAL LIKE THEIR OWN PERSONAL HERALD. LOUD AND PROUD, THIS RATING IS MEASURED IN TRUMPETS.

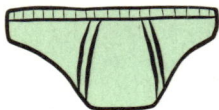

MESSINESS RATING: FARTS THAT ARE STRONG IN THIS CATEGORY DO NOT DISCRIMINATE BETWEEN SOLIDS, GASES AND LIQUIDS – THEY CAN COME IN A VARIETY OF SMELLS, SHAPES AND FORMS. THE MESSIER A FART IS, THE MORE LIKELY YOU'LL NEED A CHANGE OF PANTS, SO THIS ASPECT IS MEASURED IN PANTS.

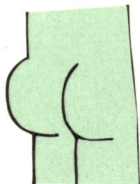

OVERALL: THIS RATING IS BASED ON A COMBINATION OF EACH OF THE ABOVE CRITERIA AS WELL AS A CERTAIN *JE NE SAIS QUOI*, WHICH COULD BE DESCRIBED AS THE GENERAL EFFECT OF THE FART. AS A FART IS NOTHING WITHOUT ITS MAKER, THE OVERALL RATING IS MEASURED IN BUMS.

THE REAL STINKERS

THESE FARTS ARE THE PINNACLE OF PUTRID. THEY'RE BOUND TO GET YOUR EYES WATERING, YOUR NOSTRILS FLARING AND YOUR GAG REFLEX, ER, FLEXING...

THE LINGERER (AKA THE HOUSE GUEST)

SMELLINESS RATING:

LOUDNESS RATING:

MESSINESS RATING:

OVERALL:

AT FIRST, THIS FART SEEMS LIKE YOUR EVERYDAY FLATULENCE. BUT WHEN, 20 MINUTES LATER, IT'S STILL THERE, YOU KNOW YOU HAVE A PROBLEM. IF YOU RELEASE ONE OF THESE IN YOUR OWN HOME THEN YOUR ONLY OPTION IS TO MOVE. EITHER IT GOES OR YOU DO, AND IT'S NOT SHIFTING!

THE STINKY HOUDINI

SMELLINESS RATING:

LOUDNESS RATING:

MESSINESS RATING:

OVERALL:

A SURREPTITIOUS RELEASE OF SILENT-BUT-DEADLY GAS INTO A CROWDED AREA. THE SECRET TO THE SUCCESS OF THIS FART IS TO TIME THE RELEASE SO THAT A QUICK ESCAPE CAN BE MADE BEFORE THE ODOUR DEVELOPS MAXIMUM STINKINESS. FAILURE TO FLEE THE VICINITY COULD LEAD TO A FATE WORSE THAN DEATH: FALLING VICTIM TO YOUR OWN NOXIOUS CLOUD.

DID YOU KNOW?

ONLY 1 PER CENT OF THE GAS THAT
MAKES UP FARTS GIVES THEM THEIR
SMELL. IT'S THE SULPHUR CONTENT
IN HYDROGEN SULPHIDE THAT GIVES
THEM THEIR UNIQUE AROMA.

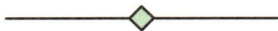

◇

THE AVERAGE PERSON FARTS BETWEEN
TEN AND TWENTY TIMES PER DAY.

EGG BARON

SMELLINESS RATING:

LOUDNESS RATING:

MESSINESS RATING:

OVERALL:

THIS ONE IS PARTICULARLY NAUSEA-INDUCING.
THE LINGERING SMELL OF ROTTEN EGGS
WILL NOT ONLY PERMEATE YOUR CLOTHES
BUT THOSE OF UNFORTUNATE BYSTANDERS.
THE ONLY WAY TO COVER UP THIS ONE
IS TO CALL CHEERILY, 'EGG SANDWICHES,
ANYONE?' AS YOU WHIP OUT A LUNCH
PLATTER FROM YOUR BACK POCKET. YUM!

AIR BISCUIT

SMELLINESS RATING:

LOUDNESS RATING:

MESSINESS RATING:

OVERALL:

THIS FART IS SO POTENT THAT YOU CAN
ALMOST HOLD IT, LIKE A BISCUIT. YOU
MIGHT NOT WANT TO DIP THIS PARTICULAR
TREAT IN YOUR TEA, THOUGH.

FART JOKES

LYING IN BED ONE NIGHT, A MAN
RELEASED A SILENT FART AND
LIFTED THE QUILT TO AIR IT OUT.

'BLIMEY, THAT STINKS!'
SHOUTED HIS WIFE.

IT MUST'VE BEEN BAD, THOUGHT
THE MAN. HIS WIFE WAS
DOWNSTAIRS AT THE TIME.

GASSY ASSASSIN

SMELLINESS RATING:

LOUDNESS RATING:

MESSINESS RATING:

OVERALL:

THIS SILENT BUT DEADLY FLUMP IS A CLASSIC. LETTING ONE OF THESE GO IS A PLEASURE, AND THE SMELLIER, THE BETTER, AS NO ONE WILL KNOW IT'S YOU, UNLESS YOU'RE CAUGHT HIGH-FIVING YOURSELF.

CULTURED FARTS

LIKE ALL THINGS, FARTS ARE NOT CREATED IN A VACUUM (THOUGH WE SOMETIMES WISH THEY WERE!). THEY ARE INFLUENCED BY THE CULTURE WE ENJOY, BE IT MUSIC, ART, FILM OR ANY OTHER FORM OF EXPRESSION. THESE EMISSIONS TRULY PUT THE 'F' IN 'ART'.

GONE WITH THE WIND

SMELLINESS RATING:

LOUDNESS RATING:

MESSINESS RATING:

OVERALL:

IF THERE WAS AN OSCARS FOR OUTSTANDING ACHIEVEMENT IN PERFORMING FARTS, THIS ONE WOULD SWEEP THE BOARD. IT STANDS THE TEST OF TIME AND DEMONSTRATES THE BEST AND WORST OF THE HUMAN CONDITION – OFTEN THE RESULT OF MIXING YOUR DRINKS AND STOPPING OFF FOR A KEBAB ON YOUR WAY HOME – SOMETHING WE MUST ALL EXPERIENCE AT LEAST ONCE IN A LIFETIME. IN THE WORDS OF MARGARET MITCHELL, 'IT WAS BETTER TO KNOW THE WORST THAN TO WONDER.'

FARTING ETIQUETTE

WHEN MINGLING AT A SOCIAL EVENT AND A SILENT FART SLIPS OUT, LEAVE ABRUPTLY AS IT HAPPENS. IT WILL TAKE A FEW SECONDS FOR THE ODOUR TO LEAVE YOUR TROUSERS. ONCE IT'S GONE, YOU CAN GET BACK TO MINGLING AND LEAVE THE FART BEHIND.

THE WIND IN THE WILLOWS

SMELLINESS RATING:

LOUDNESS RATING:

MESSINESS RATING:

OVERALL:

THE SOUNDS OF AN ENGLISH SUMMER...
DUCKS QUACKING, FROGS CROAKING, LEATHER
ON WILLOW, BUT, 'WHAT'S THAT NOISE?
IT SOUNDS LIKE A TINY TRUMPET,' SAYS
YOUR COMPANION, TO WHICH YOU REPLY,
'NO, THAT'S THE WIND IN THE WILLOWS...'

NIGHT OF THE LIVING FARTS

SMELLINESS RATING:

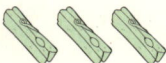

LOUDNESS RATING:

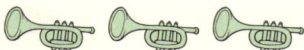

MESSINESS RATING:

OVERALL:

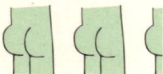

THIS FART IS THE PERFECT ACCOMPANIMENT
TO A NIGHT ON THE SOFA, A DIRTY TAKEAWAY
AND A BOX SET OF COMEDY-HORROR
FILMS, BECAUSE YOU NEVER KNOW WHEN
THE NEXT ANAL BELCH IS GOING TO STRIKE.

DID YOU KNOW?

AN AVERAGE FART IS MADE UP OF:
58 PER CENT NITROGEN
21 PER CENT HYDROGEN
9 PER CENT CARBON DIOXIDE
7 PER CENT METHANE
4 PER CENT OXYGEN
1 PER CENT HYDROGEN SULPHIDE

50 SHADES OF BROWN

SMELLINESS RATING:

LOUDNESS RATING:

MESSINESS RATING:

OVERALL:

A BODICE-RIPPING FART ONLY TO BE
RELEASED IN THE PRESENCE OF CONSENTING
ADULTS, WITH CLEAR BOUNDARIES AND
SAFE WORDS IN PLACE. IF YOUR TASTES
ARE VERY SINGULAR, THIS FART WILL SURELY
GET YOUR INNER GODDESS FARTING.

FEEL THE FORCE!

SMELLINESS RATING:

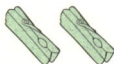

LOUDNESS RATING:

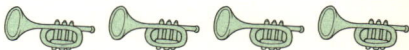

MESSINESS RATING:

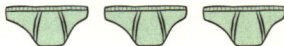

OVERALL:

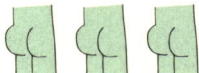

A FART THAT IS SO LOUD IT CAN BE FELT
A LONG TIME AGO, IN A GALAXY FAR,
FAR AWAY. THE PERFECT WAY TO TELL
SOMEONE, 'NO, I AM YOUR FARTER!'

FART JOKES

WHAT DO YOU CALL A PERSON
THAT NEVER FARTS IN PUBLIC?

A PRIVATE TOOTER.

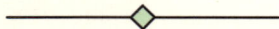

◆

WHAT'S THE DIFFERENCE BETWEEN
MOZART AND A FART?

ONE IS MUSIC TO YOUR EAR; THE
OTHER IS MUSIC FROM YOUR REAR.

BUM RAP

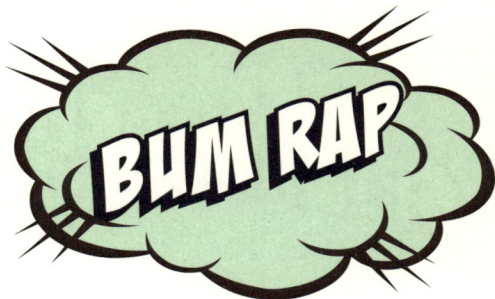

SMELLINESS RATING:

LOUDNESS RATING:

MESSINESS RATING:

OVERALL:

DO A ONE-EIGHTY WITH YOUR CAP AND
DROP YOUR WAISTBAND TO YOUR KNEES,
BECAUSE THIS TROUSER WHISTLE IS ALL
IN THE PRESENTATION. SWAGGER TO A
HIP-HOP BEAT TILL IT DROPS OUT AND
ROUND IT OFF WITH A FREESTYLE RAP.

SPINAL PARP

SMELLINESS RATING:

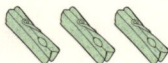

LOUDNESS RATING:

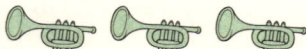

MESSINESS RATING:

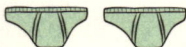

OVERALL:

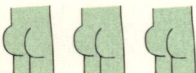

SEE, MOST FARTS GO UP TO TEN, BUT
THIS FART, THIS FART GOES UP TO
ELEVEN. THAT'S ONE FARTIER... AFTER
GETTING A WHIFF OF THIS, YOU'LL WISH
YOU JUST SMELLED THE GLOVE.

FARTING ETIQUETTE

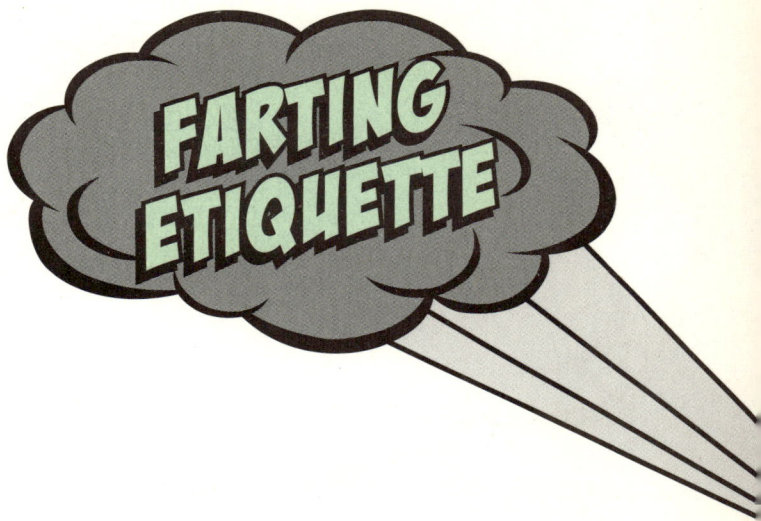

IF YOU RELEASE A STINKY EMISSION WHILST
OUT WALKING THE DOG THEN IT'S ALWAYS
FINE TO BLAME THE DOG. WITH THEIR CUTE
LITTLE TAILS AND PLAYFUL DEMEANOURS,
DOGS CAN GET AWAY WITH ANYTHING.

MUSICAL FARTS

CREATIVE FARTS COME IN MANY FORMS, BUT THESE FARTS ALL HAVE AN UNDOUBTABLE MUSICALITY, ENDEARING THEM TO THE HEARER AND LIGHTENING THE SOUL, LIKE A CHOIR OF ANGELS SINGING ON TOP OF A PARTICULARLY WHIFFY RUBBISH TIP.

TOILET TUNES

SMELLINESS RATING:

LOUDNESS RATING:

MESSINESS RATING:

OVERALL:

EVERYONE ENJOYS BUSTING A FEW TOILET
TUNES. IF YOU DISCOVER YOU HAVE AN
AUDIENCE WAITING OUTSIDE TO USE THE
CONVENIENCE, ACT LIKE YOU'VE PERFORMED
THE GIG OF YOUR LIFE AND TAKE A BOW
AS YOU MAKE YOUR EXIT. YOU COULD EVEN
OFFER A TICKET TO YOUR NEXT GIG, OR
SIGN A PIECE OF TOILET PAPER FOR THEM
- WASH YOUR HANDS FIRST THOUGH.

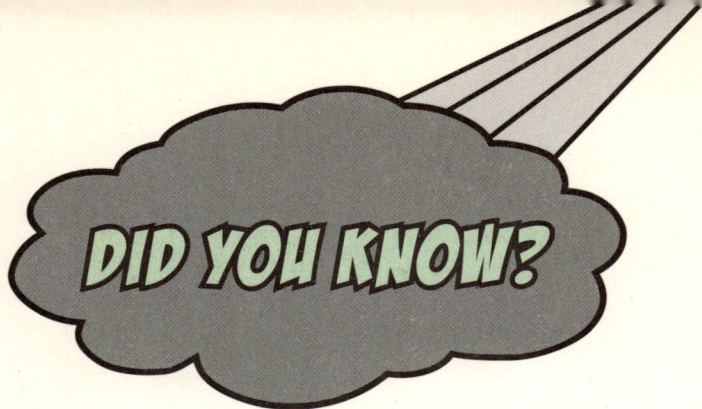

AN ANCIENT JAPANESE PIECE OF ARTWORK (OR 'FARTWORK') FROM THE EDO PERIOD, ENTITLED *HE-GASSEN* (THE FART WAR), DEPICTS MEN AND WOMEN ATTACKING EACH OTHER WITH FARTS.

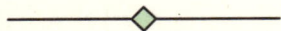

FARTING IS ACTUALLY GOOD FOR YOU! THE BACTERIA THAT PRODUCES THE GAS ALSO GENERATES VITAMINS THAT HELP TO SUPPORT OUR IMMUNE SYSTEMS.

TRUMPET CHORUS

SMELLINESS RATING: 🧷🧷🧷🧷

LOUDNESS RATING: 🎺🎺🎺🎺

MESSINESS RATING: 👙👙

OVERALL: 🍑🍑🍑🍑

THE ABILITY TO PRODUCE A MELODY FROM YOUR BOTTOM IS THE HOLY GRAIL FOR CONNOISSEURS OF ANAL WIND. WHILST MANY FARTS SOUND LIKE AN OFF-KEY TRUMPET, A TRUMPET CHORUS IS HARMONIOUS, LIKE A CHORUS OF ANGELS, BUT THEY STILL STINK!

SING THE ANAL ANTHEM

SMELLINESS RATING:

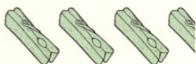

LOUDNESS RATING:

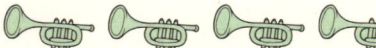

MESSINESS RATING:

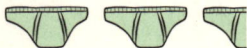

OVERALL:

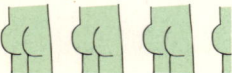

A POST-PUB FAVOURITE – WHEN YOU'RE TOO DRUNK TO SING OASIS'S GREATEST HITS, YOUR BUM CAN DO IT FOR YOU. A CHAMP-ANAL *SUPERNOVA*, IF YOU WILL.

FART JOKES

WHAT IS IT CALLED WHEN A MEMBER OF THE ARISTOCRACY FARTS?

A NOBLE GAS.

---◇---

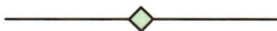

WHAT'S THE DIFFERENCE BETWEEN AN ARCHAEOLOGIST AND A FLATULIST?

ONE HAS ARTEFACTS; THE OTHER DOES FARTY ACTS.

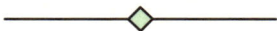

---◇---

WHY COULDN'T THE SKELETON FART IN PUBLIC?

BECAUSE HE HAD NO GUTS.

FROG CHORUS

SMELLINESS RATING:

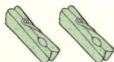

LOUDNESS RATING:

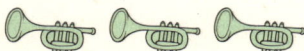

MESSINESS RATING:

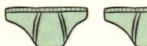

OVERALL:

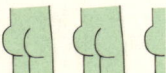

THIS IS THE BARITONE OF FARTS –
A SOUND SO DEEP THAT YOU CAN FEEL
THE FLOOR VIBRATE. LIKE OPERA SINGING,
IT TAKES YEARS TO HONE THIS SKILL AND
PRODUCE SUCH SILKY TONES – MANY
HAVE TRIED AND MOST HAVE ENDED
UP DESTROYING THEIR UNDERWEAR.

THE ASCENDER

SMELLINESS RATING:

LOUDNESS RATING:

MESSINESS RATING:

OVERALL:

NAMED FOR ITS TONE, THE ASCENDER STARTS
OFF AS A DEEP, GUTTURAL RUMBLE, BUT
RISES IN PITCH TO END AS A SQUEAK – LIKE
AIR BEING RELEASED FROM A BALLOON.
IT CAN BE ACHIEVED THROUGH PRECISION
MOVEMENT OF THE BUTT CHEEKS, EXPERT
CHOICE IN SEATING MATERIAL, OR SIMPLY
THE FART GODS SMILING ON YOU THAT
DAY. FOR OPTIMUM IMPACT, THE FART
SHOULD LAST FOR AT LEAST 3 SECONDS.

FART JOKES

'I HAD AN INTERVIEW YESTERDAY FOR A NEW JOB DISTRIBUTING LEAFLETS ON FLATULENCE AWARENESS.

IT WAS ALL GOING SO WELL UNTIL I LET ONE RIP.'

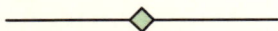

◇

'I DIDN'T FART IN FRONT OF MY WIFE UNTIL AFTER WE WERE MARRIED.

IT WAS A HUGE RELIEF FOR ME, BUT I DON'T THINK THE WEDDING PARTY WAS IMPRESSED.'

BROWN BRASS CHOIR

SMELLINESS RATING:

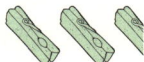

LOUDNESS RATING:

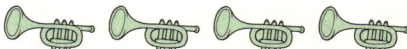

MESSINESS RATING:

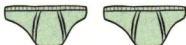

OVERALL:

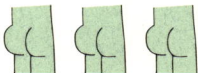

THE ROUSING SOUND OF A BRASS
BAND EMANATING FROM YOUR NETHER
REGIONS WILL MAKE YOU MISTY-EYED...
EVEN IF YOU WEREN'T BROUGHT UP
IN A SMALL COAL-MINING TOWN.

PARPSICHORD

SMELLINESS RATING:

LOUDNESS RATING:

MESSINESS RATING:

OVERALL:

AS MELODIOUS AS IT IS MALODOROUS
– A SOUND TO DELIGHT THE AURAL AND
THE ANAL, ERM, BITS. THIS ONE WILL
REALLY IMPRESS THE FUTURE MOTHER-IN-
LAW WHEN YOU'RE ASKED TO PERFORM
A POST-SUNDAY LUNCH RECITAL.

DID YOU KNOW?

IN 2011, THE MALAWI GOVERNMENT INTRODUCED NEW LEGISLATION INTENDED TO PROHIBIT FOULING OF THE AIR. JOURNALISTS INTERPRETED THIS AS A BAN ON BREAKING WIND AND THE NEWS WENT GLOBAL, WITH MALAWI'S MINISTER OF JUSTICE INITIALLY BACKING UP THE CLAIMS, THEN LATER RETRACTING HIS COMMENTS.

FART ATTACKS

WITH GREAT FART POWER COMES GREAT RESPONSIBILITY, WHICH THESE FARTS BLATANTLY FLOUT, UTILISING NEFARIOUS BUTT GAS TO INFLICT HARM ON OTHERS. TUT TUT.

MAGIC CUPCAKE

SMELLINESS RATING:

LOUDNESS RATING:

MESSINESS RATING:

OVERALL:

AS GIFTS GO, THIS ONE STINKS! CUP
YOUR HAND BENEATH YOUR REAR END
TO 'CATCH' YOUR FART, THEN QUICKLY
FLING IT AT THE DESIRED RECIPIENT. THEY
WON'T FORGET THIS GIFT IN A HURRY!

FART JOKES

A MAN WALKS INTO A JEWELLERY
SHOP AND BENDS DOWN TO LOOK AT
A FINE GOLD WATCH. AS HE DOES SO,
MUCH TO HIS SURPRISE, HE BREAKS
WIND. A SHOP ASSISTANT GOES UP
TO HIM AND ASKS IF SHE CAN BE OF
ANY HELP. 'YES,' REPLIES THE MAN.
'HOW MUCH FOR THAT WATCH?'

'SIR, IF YOU FARTED JUST LOOKING
AT IT, YOU'LL POO YOURSELF
WHEN YOU HEAR THE PRICE.'

DUTCH OVEN

SMELLINESS RATING:

LOUDNESS RATING:

MESSINESS RATING:

OVERALL:

THE OLD FARTING-IN-BED-AND-INSISTING-YOUR-LOVER-BATHES-IN-YOUR-SCENT-BY-INVITING-THEM-UNDER-THE-COVERS TRICK. A CLASSIC FART, THOUGH NOT RECOMMENDED IF YOU'RE TRYING TO IMPRESS A NEW LOVE, UNLESS THEY LIKE THAT SORT OF THING.

THE 'I DROPPED MY PENCIL'

SMELLINESS RATING:

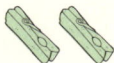

LOUDNESS RATING:

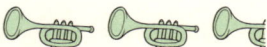

MESSINESS RATING:

OVERALL:

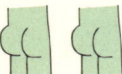

A DASTARDLY WEAPONISATION OF YOUR DIGESTIVE GASES; SIMPLY WALK PAST YOUR SEATED VICTIM, 'ACCIDENTALLY' DROP YOUR PENCIL/DIDGERIDOO/POT PLANT (WHICHEVER BEST SUITS THE SITUATION), BEND OVER TO PICK IT UP AND BAM, DIRECT HIT! BE WARNED BEFORE USING THIS FART: THE ATTACK IS SO BLATANT THAT RETALIATION WILL ALMOST CERTAINLY BE FORTHCOMING, SO A CLEAN GETAWAY IS NECESSARY.

FARTING ETIQUETTE

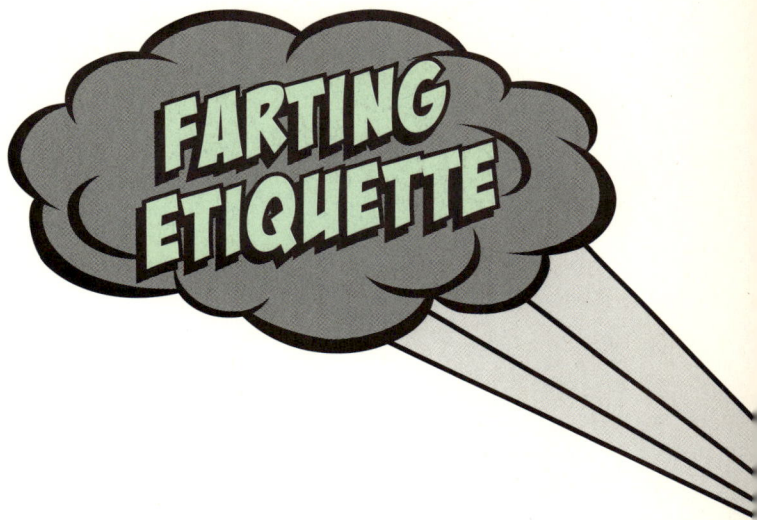

IF YOU FEEL A FART APPROACHING AND
YOU'RE IN BED WITH YOUR PARTNER, THEN
YOU WILL NEED TO ASSESS WHETHER
TO GO AHEAD WITH IT. WILL YOUR OTHER
HALF APPRECIATE THE SENTIMENT? IF,
HOWEVER, YOU ARE IN BED ALONE THEN
FEEL FREE TO FART THE NIGHT AWAY.

THE DIRTY PROTEST

SMELLINESS RATING:

LOUDNESS RATING:

MESSINESS RATING:

OVERALL:

A TOXIC COCKTAIL OF SPITE AND
METHANE. TYPICALLY RELEASED DURING
PERIODS OF INTENSE ANNOYANCE
AND IRRITATION, SUCH AS DURING A
PRETENTIOUS *AVANT-GARDE* MODERN
DANCE PERFORMANCE OR A SLIDESHOW
OF YOUR CO-WORKER'S HOLIDAY SNAPS.

TRAVEL FARTS

BY AIR, BY RAIL, BY ROAD AND BY BIKE, YOU CAN TRY TO ESCAPE THESE FARTS, BUT THEY'LL ALWAYS BE WITH YOU ON YOUR JOURNEY.

PRESSURE RELEASE VALVE

SMELLINESS RATING:

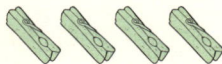

LOUDNESS RATING:

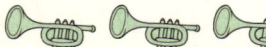

MESSINESS RATING:

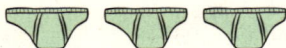

OVERALL:

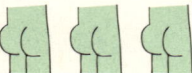

A FART YOU'RE MOST LIKELY TO ENCOUNTER
AFTER A 12-HOUR COACH JOURNEY
WITHOUT A WORKING TOILET ON BOARD
AND WITH NO REST STOPS. THERE'S ONLY
SO LONG YOU CAN HOLD YOUR BOWELS
BEFORE SOMETHING'S GOT TO GIVE.
SUMMONING OTHER-WORLDLY POWERS,
YOUR BODY INFUSES THE ESSENCE OF YOUR
WITHHELD MONSTER POO INTO A FART.
THAT'LL TEACH YOUR FELLOW TRAVELLERS
TO FALL ASLEEP ON YOUR SHOULDER
AND KICK THE BACK OF YOUR CHAIR.

DID YOU KNOW?

THE REASON PEOPLE ARE LESS
BOTHERED BY THEIR OWN FARTS THAN
OTHER PEOPLE'S IS SIMPLY THAT THEY
BECOME ACCUSTOMED TO THEM.
EVERY DIGESTIVE SYSTEM IS DIFFERENT
AND THEREFORE EVERYONE'S FARTS
HAVE A SLIGHTLY DIFFERENT ODOUR.

COMMUTE TOOT

SMELLINESS RATING:

LOUDNESS RATING:

MESSINESS RATING:

OVERALL:

THE ACT OF PASSING WIND ON A BUSY
COMMUTER TRAIN. WHEN YOU'RE SO
SQUASHED IN YOUR FEET NO LONGER TOUCH
THE FLOOR, IT'S A PRETTY SAFE BET THAT
NO ONE WILL KNOW IT WAS YOU. JUST
MAKE SURE YOU KEEP A STRAIGHT FACE.

TURDULANCE

SMELLINESS RATING:

LOUDNESS RATING:

MESSINESS RATING:

OVERALL:

THIS IS WHAT HAPPENS WHEN YOU HOLD
IN YOUR FLATUS FOR TOO LONG ON A
LONG-HAUL FLIGHT BECAUSE YOU DON'T
WANT TO USE THOSE HORRIBLE PLANE
TOILETS. ADOPT THE BRACE POSITION AND
ENSURE YOUR SEATBELT IS FASTENED.

FART JOKES

TEACHER: JAMES, PLEASE USE THE WORD 'DEFINITELY' IN A SENTENCE.

JAMES: YES, SIR. SHOULD FARTS BE LUMPY, SIR?

TEACHER: OF COURSE NOT, JAMES, NOW ANSWER THE QUESTION.

JAMES: YES, SIR. I HAVE DEFINITELY POOED MY PANTS.

PARPCYCLE

SMELLINESS RATING:

LOUDNESS RATING:

MESSINESS RATING:

OVERALL:

THERE'S NOTHING LIKE A BRISK BIKE RIDE TO REINVIGORATE THE SENSES, GET YOUR BLOOD FLOWING AND BREATHE IN SOME FRESH AIR. BUT WHAT TO DO IF YOU FIND YOURSELF HALFWAY UP A MONSTER OF A HILL, QUICKLY RUNNING OUT OF STEAM? LET ONE RIP AND PARP YOUR WAY TO THE TOP OF THE HILL. SO MUCH FOR THAT FRESH AIR...

DIGESTIVE JUSTICE

THERE'S A PHRASE IN COMPUTING WHICH GOES 'GARBAGE IN, GARBAGE OUT'. THIS PHRASE CAN BE APPLIED WITH AS MUCH ACCURACY TO FARTING. AS YOU WILL REAP WHAT YOU SOW, YOU WILL FART WHAT YOU EAT.

AIR ON A G-STRING

SMELLINESS RATING:

LOUDNESS RATING:

MESSINESS RATING:

OVERALL:

A WEDDING FAVOURITE, BUT FOR ALL
THE WRONG REASONS. WHO WOULD
HAVE THOUGHT CONSUMING 30 EGG
VOL-AU-VENTS AND A FULL CASE OF
LAGER COULD HAVE SUCH AN EFFECT?

DID YOU KNOW?

THE FARTS OF FEMALE SOUTHERN PINE BEETLES CONTAIN A PHEROMONE CALLED FRONTALIN, WHICH THEY USE TO CALL OTHER MEMBERS OF THEIR SPECIES. THE PHEROMONE IS ESPECIALLY ATTRACTIVE TO MALES OF THE SPECIES.

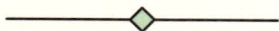

———◆———

STUDIES HAVE SHOWN THAT SMELLING HYDROGEN SULPHIDE (THE SUBSTANCE THAT MAKES FARTS SMELL) COULD HAVE A HEALTH BENEFIT, REDUCING THE RISK OF STROKES, HEART ATTACKS, CANCER, ARTHRITIS AND DEMENTIA.

SILENT STINK

SMELLINESS RATING:

LOUDNESS RATING:

MESSINESS RATING:

OVERALL:

IT'S DOUBTFUL THAT EVEN YOU WILL FORESEE
THE ARRIVAL OF THIS PARTICULAR POPPER,
AS IT SLIPS OUT LIKE THE DEVIL IN VELVET
TROUSERS. 'OH, I WISH I HADN'T EATEN THAT
FRIDGE PACK OF BEANS ALL TO MYSELF!'
YOU MIGHT SAY, AND YOU'D BE RIGHT.

THE FESTIVE FART

SMELLINESS RATING:

LOUDNESS RATING:

MESSINESS RATING:

OVERALL:

WE ALL LIKE TO INDULGE IN A SPROUT OR TEN
AT YULETIDE, BUT THE RESULTANT CAROLLING
THAT WARBLES OUT OF YOUR REAR IS SADLY
NOT SO DESIRABLE. ONLY LET THIS ONE
GO WHEN YOU'RE SURROUNDED BY PEOPLE
WHO REALLY LOVE YOU, AND TRY TO HOLD
IT IN DURING THE QUEEN'S SPEECH UNLESS
YOU CAN FART THE NATIONAL ANTHEM.

FART JOKES

MATTHEW GOES TO HIS GRANDPARENTS' HOUSE FOR DINNER EVERY SUNDAY. AFTER A DELICIOUS MEAL OF CAULIFLOWER CHEESE, BROCCOLI AND LAMB, MATTHEW FEELS A GURGLE IN HIS STOMACH AND KNOWS HE HAS TO FART. HE SLYLY LIFTS A BUTTOCK OFF THE SEAT AND TRIES TO LET ONE OUT QUIETLY, BUT FAILS – THE PARP IS NOT OVERLY LOUD, BUT CERTAINLY AUDIBLE. STRAIGHT AWAY, MATTHEW'S GRANDAD LOOKS AT THE FAMILY DOG, SITTING AT MATTHEW'S FEET, AND SCOLDS 'BAILEY!' DELIGHTED, BUT STILL FEELING UNCOMFORTABLE, MATTHEW LETS OUT ANOTHER FART, THIS TIME LOUDER. AGAIN, HIS GRANDAD LOOKS AT THE DOG AND SCOLDS HIM. WITH RECKLESS ABANDON, MATTHEW ATTEMPTS TO BE RID OF ALL OF HIS GAS, AND LETS OUT A HUGE HONKING FART. 'BAILEY!' SHOUTS MATTHEW'S GRANDAD. 'GET AWAY FROM THAT FILTHY BOY BEFORE HE POOS ON YOU!'

FARTNADO

SMELLINESS RATING:

LOUDNESS RATING:

MESSINESS RATING:

OVERALL:

EVERYONE HAS A PARTICULAR FOOD THAT
THEY SHOULDN'T GO WITHIN TEN FEET OF
(MINE'S ONIONS IN CASE YOU WERE
WONDERING) AND SHOULD A MERE MORSEL
OF SAID FOOD PASS YOUR LIPS – SOMETIMES
THROUGH NO FAULT OF YOUR OWN – ALL
HELL BREAKS LOOSE. IT'S AS THOUGH THE
GREAT STORM FROM *THE WIZARD OF OZ*
IS SWIRLING IN YOUR LOWER BOWEL, ONLY
THERE WON'T BE A YELLOW BRICK ROAD AT
THE END OF IT, MORE LIKE A BROWN ONE.

THE COLON-IAL

SMELLINESS RATING:

LOUDNESS RATING:

MESSINESS RATING:

OVERALL:

THE BODY'S REACTION TO A SEVERE CHANGE IN DIET, USUALLY EXPERIENCED ON HOLIDAY IN A FAR-FLUNG EXOTIC LOCATION. IF PRONE TO THIS REACTION, YOU'RE IN A NO-WIN SITUATION; YOU'RE EITHER GURNING AND FARTING FOR YOUR WHOLE HOLIDAY OR YOU'RE THE UNADVENTUROUS TOURIST WHO KEEPS ASKING RESTAURANTS IF THEY SERVE CHIPS.

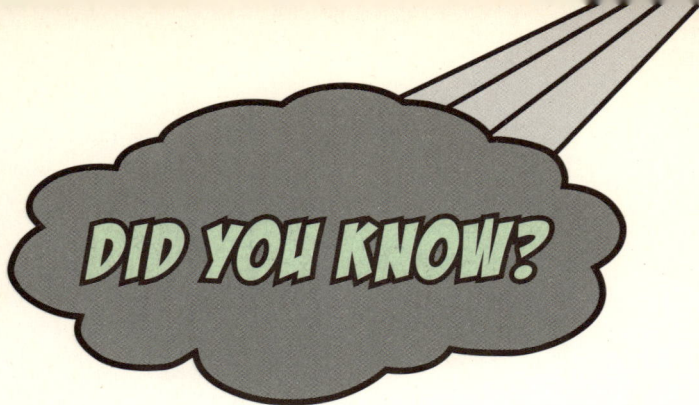

THE WORD 'FART' HAS BEEN AROUND FOR A VERY LONG TIME, AND WAS PRESENT IN MANY DIFFERENT INDO-EUROPEAN LANGUAGES. ANOTHER WORD FOR FARTING THAT HAS BEEN LOST THROUGH TIME IS 'FIST', WHICH, THROUGH A DEROGATORY TERM FOR LAPDOGS, WE GET THE WORD 'FEISTY'.

DANGER FARTS

FARTS FOR THE RISK-TAKERS OF THE WORLD,
THE TRUE MAVERICKS WHO ARE WILLING TO
TAKE THEIR OWN LIVES (AND THE LIVES OF
THOSE AROUND THEM) INTO THEIR HANDS
(OR, MORE ACCURATELY, BUTT CHEEKS) AND
GAMBLE IT ALL ON THAT ONE MAJESTIC PARP.

RING-STINGER

SMELLINESS RATING:

LOUDNESS RATING:

MESSINESS RATING:

OVERALL:

HOT WINDS DOWN BELOW CAN LEAD TO THIS COMPLAINT, AND THE RING-STINGER PARTICULARLY SMARTS. BE PREPARED FOR THIS ONE AFTER A HOT CURRY OR SPICY MEXICAN FOOD BY PUTTING A FEW ROLLS OF TOILET PAPER IN THE FRIDGE.

FART JOKES

A WOMAN WALKS INTO A CAFE AND SITS DOWN. AS SHE DOES SO, SHE LETS OUT A MASSIVE FART, CAUSING THE MAN SAT BEHIND HER TO CHUCKLE HEARTILY. EMBARRASSED, THE WOMAN SNAPS AT HIM, 'STOP THAT!'

'I COULD TRY,' THE MAN REPLIES, 'BUT I DON'T KNOW WHICH WAY IT WENT!'

PEAKY BLINDER

SMELLINESS RATING:

LOUDNESS RATING:

MESSINESS RATING:

OVERALL:

THIS FART SHOULD CARRY A HEALTH
WARNING AND MUST NOT BE ATTEMPTED
WITHIN A CONFINED SPACE, UNLESS YOU
WISH TO APE THE DEFENCE MECHANISM
OF A SKUNK AGAINST YOUR FOE, AS THE
SMELL WILL RENDER THEM TEMPORARILY
BLIND AS THEY PULL DOWN THEIR FLAT
CAP TO COVER THEIR NOSTRILS.

FLAMETHROWER

SMELLINESS RATING:

LOUDNESS RATING:

MESSINESS RATING:

OVERALL:

LIGHTING A FART IS A RITE OF PASSAGE – THE ANAL PASSAGE! TO AVOID A TERRIBLE ESCALATION, THIS FART SHOULD NOT BE ATTEMPTED NEAR ANY FLAMMABLE UPHOLSTERY OR IN FORESTS DURING DRY SEASONS.

FARTING ETIQUETTE

IN THE EVENT OF A SILENT FART WHERE
IT'S DIFFICULT TO ESCAPE, WAIT FOR
20 SECONDS AFTER SMELLING YOUR OWN
FART. AFTER THIS TIME, LOOK AROUND
DISGUSTEDLY AS IF TO SAY, 'WHO FARTED?'
THE DELAY WILL MEAN THAT THOSE SITTING
NEAR YOU WILL THINK THE OFFENDING SMELL
REACHED THEM BEFORE YOU, THEREBY
CLEARING YOUR NAME AS THE CULPRIT.
NB IF YOUR CHAIR HAS A SOLID BOTTOM,
RATHER THAN HOLES OR MESH, ENSURE YOU
ADD A FEW SECONDS ON TO THE DELAY
AS THE FART WILL NOT EXIT SO EASILY.

BLOW THE HOUSE DOWN

SMELLINESS RATING:

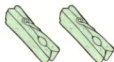

LOUDNESS RATING:

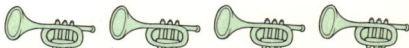

MESSINESS RATING:

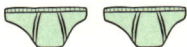

OVERALL:

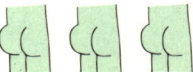

NOT TO BE PERFORMED ON A FAULT
LINE – IMAGINE THE CARNAGE – AND IT'S
MOST UNLIKELY THAT YOU'LL BE ABLE
TO CLAIM IT ON INSURANCE, UNLESS
YOU CAN CONVINCE YOUR BROKER
THAT A FART IS AN ACT OF GOD.

RECREATIONAL FARTING

YOU KNOW THE SAYING: ALL REST AND NO PLAY MAKES JACK A DULL FARTER (THAT'S DEFINITELY HOW IT GOES). THESE FARTS ARE FOR THE JESTERS AND PLAYFUL TRICKSTERS, FARTING WITH RECKLESS ABANDON AND GLEE.

PULL MY FINGER

SMELLINESS RATING:

LOUDNESS RATING:

MESSINESS RATING:

OVERALL:

OH GO ON, YOU KNOW YOU WANT TO. THAT OLD PARTY TRICK OF FARTING ON COMMAND IS A LIFE SKILL – PERHAPS WORTHY OF GOING ON THE CV.

FART JOKES

TWO BROTHERS ARE SITTING
ON THE SOFA WATCHING TV.

THE YOUNGEST SUDDENLY GRIMACES.
'HAVE YOU FARTED?' HE ASKS.

'ME?! NO!'

'I BET YOU TWENTY QUID YOU HAVE!'

SMILING SMUGLY, THE ELDER
SHOWS HIS BROTHER HIS PANTS
AND SAYS, 'I TOLD YOU IT WASN'T
A FART, TWENTY QUID PLEASE!'

PULL MY LEG

SMELLINESS RATING:

LOUDNESS RATING:

MESSINESS RATING:

OVERALL:

THIS IS UNIVERSITY-LEVEL FARTING. IT'S ONE
THAT WILL MAKE A LASTING IMPRESSION
AT ANY SOCIAL EVENT, ESPECIALLY IF YOU
DROP THIS DEVIL AT FRESHERS' WEEK.
PREPARE FOR IT WITH THE STANDARD
STUDENT FARE OF CORNED BEEF AND
BEANS, LOOSEN UP WITH SOME LUNGES
AND WEAR BAGGY CLOTHING. YOU LEGEND!

YOGA FART

SMELLINESS RATING:

LOUDNESS RATING:

MESSINESS RATING:

OVERALL:

IT'S AN OCCUPATIONAL HAZARD WHEN
YOU'RE DOING THE DOWNWARD DOG, THE
TREE, OR THE BABY POSE, YOU RELAX AND
YOU HAVE TO LET ONE GO! THAT TINY SQUEAK
BETWEEN THE CHEEKS SEEMS TO ECHO
AROUND THE STUDIO, BUT FEAR NOT,
NO ONE WILL KNOW IT'S YOU, UNLESS
YOU'RE NEAR A NAKED FLAME!

STUDIES HAVE SUGGESTED THAT HERRING COMMUNICATE BY FARTING. THE NOISE, DESCRIBED BY RESEARCHERS AS BEING LIKE A HIGH-PITCHED RASPBERRY, IS MOSTLY USED AT NIGHT WHEN THE FISH ARE IN A HIGH-DENSITY SHOAL.

FART TENNIS

SMELLINESS RATING:

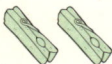

LOUDNESS RATING:

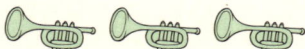

MESSINESS RATING:

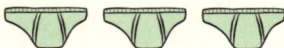

OVERALL:

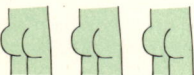

A GAME TO BE PLAYED WITH
YOUR LOVER UNDER THE COVERS,
BUT WATCH FOR THOSE POWER
SERVES AS YOU MIGHT SEE
MORE THAN CHALK DUST!

FLASH SMOG

SMELLINESS RATING:

LOUDNESS RATING:

MESSINESS RATING:

OVERALL:

A FLASH MOB OF FARTERS, TYPICALLY
ORGANISED VIA SOCIAL MEDIA
PLATFORMS SUCH AS FARTR, FARTBOOK
OR PARPCHAT. IF THE CROWD IS ABLE
TO DISPERSE BEFORE THE SMELL DOES,
YOU KNOW IT'S BEEN A SUCCESS.

FART JOKES

PATIENT: DOCTOR, YOU'VE GOT TO HELP ME, I CAN'T STOP FARTING!

DOCTOR: THAT'S QUITE A PROBLEM, DO TELL ME MORE.

PATIENT: WELL, THEY DON'T SMELL AND THEY'RE NOT NOISY, BUT I'M FARTING ALL THE TIME. I'VE FARTED ALMOST CONTINUOUSLY SINCE I'VE BEEN IN YOUR OFFICE.

DOCTOR: OK. I THINK I KNOW EXACTLY WHAT YOU NEED.

PATIENT: REALLY? SOMETHING TO STOP ME FARTING?

DOCTOR: NO. IT'LL CLEAR UP YOUR SINUSES AND YOU'LL NEED A HEARING TEST. IT STINKS IN HERE AND I COULD BARELY HEAR YOU OVER THE FARTS.

HISTORICAL FARTS

THESE FARTS HAVE BEEN HANDED DOWN
THROUGH THE GENERATIONS, FROM
PARENT TO CHILD. THEY TRULY CONNECT
US TO OUR PARPING HERITAGE AND TAKE
US BACK TO A TIME WHEN LIFE WAS
SIMPLE AND FARTS WERE STINKY.

GUSTY GUSSET

SMELLINESS RATING:

LOUDNESS RATING:

MESSINESS RATING:

OVERALL:

EVEN ENGLISH ROSES IN COSTUME
DRAMAS SUFFER FROM DRAUGHTY
DERRIÈRES. IF YOU THOUGHT THE
SWOONING WAS CAUSED BY THE ARRIVAL
OF MR PONSONBY-DARCY-HAVELOCK ON
A WHITE CHARGER, YOU ARE MISTAKEN.
IT'S THE NOXIOUS FARTS THAT GET
TRAPPED IN THE ACRES OF TAFFETA
THAT KNOCK THEM OUT!

DID YOU KNOW?

FART LIGHTING (ALSO KNOWN AS FLATUS IGNITION OR PYROFLATULENCE) IS THE PROCESS WHEREBY AN INDIVIDUAL HOLDS AN OPEN FLAME NEAR THE FART EXIT ZONE AND PRODUCES A 'BLUE ANGEL' ON EXPULSION. THIS NAME COMES FROM GASES PRODUCED IN THE COLON WHICH TURN BLUE UPON IGNITION. BEWARE THOUGH; THIS CAN BE DANGEROUS IF IT GOES WRONG AS EVIDENCED BY MANY A YOUTUBE VIDEO.

REAR ADMIRAL

SMELLINESS RATING:

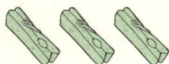

LOUDNESS RATING:

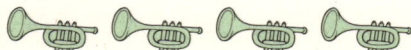

MESSINESS RATING:

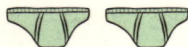

OVERALL:

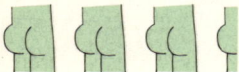

MAKE SURE YOU STAND TO ATTENTION
WHEN YOU BLOW THIS BUTT BUGLE – A MOST
STATELY AND UPSTANDING FART. EVEN
ADMIRAL NELSON HIMSELF USED THIS AS A
CALL TO ARMS AT THE BATTLE OF TRAFALGAR.

FART-GATE

SMELLINESS RATING:

LOUDNESS RATING:

MESSINESS RATING:

OVERALL:

THE SORT OF FART THAT COULD BRING DOWN A GOVERNMENT. A FART HEARD AROUND THE WORLD. A FART THAT COULD ONLY BE DENIED BY THE PHRASE 'I DID NOT HAVE CULINARY RELATIONS WITH THAT BURRITO!'

FART JOKES

AN OLD COUPLE ARE AT THEIR LOCAL CHURCH, AS THEY ARE EVERY SUNDAY MORNING. MIDWAY THROUGH THE SERVICE, THE HUSBAND LEANS OVER AND WHISPERS TO HIS WIFE, 'DON'T TELL ANYONE BUT I JUST FARTED. IT WAS SILENT THOUGH. WHAT SHOULD I DO?'

TO WHICH SHE REPLIES, 'PUT A NEW BATTERY IN YOUR HEARING AID.'

THE TOMB OF TOOT-ANKHAMUN

SMELLINESS RATING:

LOUDNESS RATING:

MESSINESS RATING:

OVERALL:

RELEASE YOUR SPHINX-TER AND
LET OUT A FART THAT THE
PHARAOHS THEMSELVES WOULD
HAVE BEEN PROUD OF.

BLAZING SADDLES

SMELLINESS RATING:

LOUDNESS RATING:

MESSINESS RATING:

OVERALL:

A HOT, FIERY FART USUALLY EXPERIENCED
AFTER A HARD DAY OF ROUNDING UP CATTLE
AND EATING REFRIED BEANS. YOU MAY
NEED TO GIVE YOUR CHAPS AND JEANS A
BIT OF AN AIRING OUT AFTER THIS ONE.

FARTING ETIQUETTE

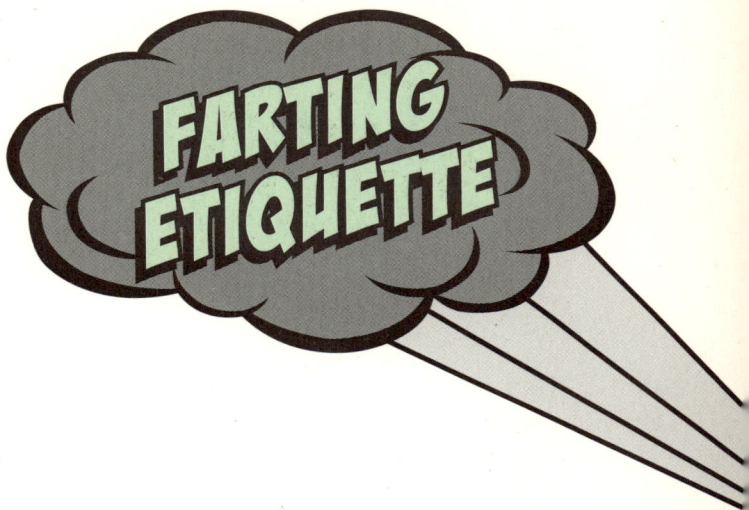

A TRULY MAGNIFICENT SITUATION TO LET ONE GO IS WHILST SKYDIVING. IF YOU'RE A CAPABLE ENOUGH PARACHUTIST THAT YOU'RE ABLE TO DO A SOLO JUMP, THEN YOU'RE FREE TO LET ONE FLY AND THE FART TRAIL WILL QUICKLY DISPERSE BEHIND YOU AS YOU HURTLE TO THE EARTH. IF YOU HAVE AN INSTRUCTOR STRAPPED TO YOUR BACK, HOPE THAT THEY LIKE YOU ENOUGH TO STILL PULL THE CHUTE AFTER YOU'VE FARTED ON THEIR CROTCH...

THE ABRABUM LINCOLN

SMELLINESS RATING:

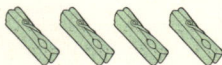

LOUDNESS RATING:

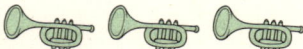

MESSINESS RATING:

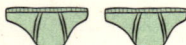

OVERALL:

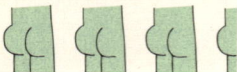

FOUR SCORE AND SEVEN CANS OF
BEANS AGO, YOU BROUGHT FORTH IN YOUR
DIGESTIVE SYSTEM A NEW ODOUR, CONCEIVED
IN GLUTTONY AND DEDICATED TO THE
PROPOSITION THAT ALL FARTS ARE CREATED
EQUALLY SMELLY. PULL YOUR STOVEPIPE HAT
DOWN TIGHT AND PRAY FOR EMANCIPATION.

MINI FARTS

THESE FARTS ARE TESTAMENT TO THE FACT
THAT GOOD THINGS DO COME IN SMALL
PACKAGES, BECAUSE IT'S NOT THE SIZE
OF THE FART, IT'S WHAT YOU DO WITH IT.

FUN-SIZE FLATULENCE

SMELLINESS RATING:

LOUDNESS RATING:

MESSINESS RATING:

OVERALL:

PERFECT TO PINCH OFF WHEN YOU DON'T HAVE TIME FOR THE LUSH, SELF-INDULGENT FART YOU'RE LONGING FOR. THE FART OF CHOICE FOR HIGH-POWERED BUSINESS PEOPLE, BUSY WAITSTAFF AND ANYBODY WHO CAN'T CATCH A MINUTE TO CUT THE CHEESE.

FART JOKES

WHAT DID THE PRIEST SAY BEFORE
HE FLUSHED THE TOILET?

HOLY CRAP!

WHY SHOULD YOU NEVER
FART IN CHURCH?

BECAUSE YOU HAVE TO STAY
SEATED IN YOUR PEW.

WHAT DO YOU CALL A FART IN GERMAN?

FARFROMPOOPIN!

POCKET PARP

SMELLINESS RATING:

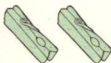

LOUDNESS RATING:

MESSINESS RATING:

OVERALL:

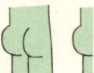

IT'S THE LITTLE THINGS IN LIFE THAT
MEAN THE MOST – THE FIRST FLOWER
OF SPRING, A SMILE FROM A BABY...
A TEENSY LITTLE POCKET PARP AS
YOU ROUSE FROM YOUR SLUMBER –
IT'S ALMOST LIKE YOUR SPHINCTER IS
SAYING A CHEERY GOOD MORNING.

SNEAKY SQUEAK

SMELLINESS RATING:

LOUDNESS RATING:

MESSINESS RATING:

OVERALL:

'WAS THAT A MOUSE?'

'WHY, YES.' THE SNEAKY SQUEAK IS A
VERSATILE TRUMP, AND ONE THAT CAN
BE DISGUISED WITH MINIMUM FUSS AT
MOST SOCIAL OCCASIONS, APART FROM
SNOOKER TOURNAMENTS WHERE YOU
JUST HAVE TO HOLD YOUR HAND UP.

DID YOU KNOW?

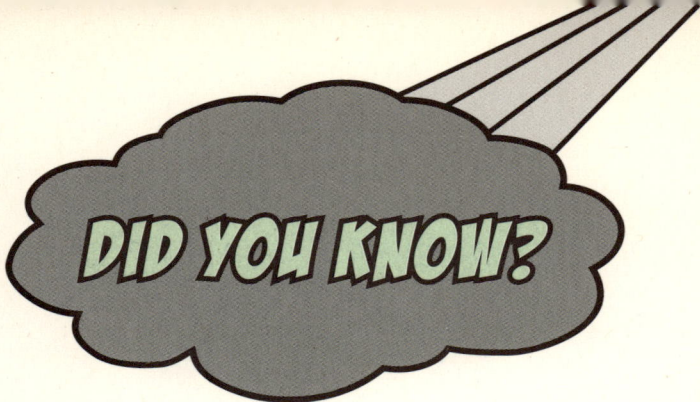

ON AVERAGE, A PERSON FARTS
AROUND 15 TIMES A DAY, AND
MOST OF THESE WILL HAPPEN WHILE
SLEEPING. THE TOTAL VOLUME OF GAS
PRODUCED IS 500–1,500 MILLILITRES.

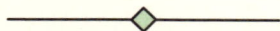

◇

FARTS HAVE BEEN MEASURED
TO TRAVEL AT SPEEDS OF
UP TO 10 FEET PER SECOND,
OR 7 MILES PER HOUR.

SQUEAKY FLOORBOARD

SMELLINESS RATING:

LOUDNESS RATING:

MESSINESS RATING:

OVERALL:

A FAVOURITE AMONG ESTATE AGENTS – AND
IF IT'S PARTICULARLY PUNGENT YOU CAN
SAY THE DRAINS MIGHT NEED LOOKING AT.

THE SOUND AND THE FURY

GET OUT THOSE EAR DEFENDERS AND TELL YOUR GRANNY TO TURN DOWN HER HEARING AID, THESE ARE THE FARTS THAT REALLY PUSH THE DECIBELS. FART LOUD AND FART PROUD!

THAR SHE BLOWS

SMELLINESS RATING:

LOUDNESS RATING:

MESSINESS RATING:

OVERALL:

THE GRANDADDY OF FARTS, AND
ONE THAT'S USUALLY PERFORMED BY
GRANDADS AND GRANDMAS. THEY'RE
SOUND ASLEEP ON THE SOFA AFTER A
BIG LUNCH, AND BEFORE TOO LONG THEY
START TO SNORE FROM BOTH ENDS.

FART JOKES

**WHAT IS THE SHARPEST
THING IN THE WORLD?**

A FART; IT GOES THROUGH YOUR PANTS
AND DOESN'T EVEN LEAVE A HOLE.

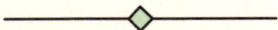

**WHAT DO YOU GET IF YOU EAT
LOADS AND LOADS OF ONIONS
AND BAKED BEANS?**

TEAR GAS.

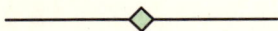

**WHAT DID THE MAXI-PAD
SAY TO THE FART?**

YOU ARE THE WIND BENEATH MY WINGS.

TROUSER COUGH

SMELLINESS RATING:

LOUDNESS RATING:

MESSINESS RATING:

OVERALL:

LIKE A LITTLE YAPPY DOG, BUT WITH NO
DOG IN SIGHT, THIS ONE IS PERSISTENT.
DISGUISE IT BY LOOKING AROUND YOU
AND CALLING OUT, 'BARNABY, COME HERE
YOU NAUGHTY DOG!' IT MIGHT WORK.

SPHINCTER SONG

SMELLINESS RATING:

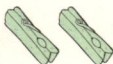

LOUDNESS RATING:

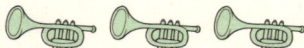

MESSINESS RATING:

OVERALL:

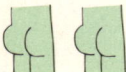

THIS IS A LOVE SONG FROM YOUR BOTTOM. FOR TRUE MASTERS, A KEY CHANGE FOR THE LAST CHORUS WILL REALLY TUG AT THE HEARTSTRINGS.

MAGGOTS HAVE LONG BEEN USED FOR CLEANING WOUNDS DUE TO THEM EATING ONLY DEAD, NOT LIVING, TISSUE, BUT NOW THE MEDICAL APPLICATION OF THE FLATULENCE OF MAGGOTS IS BEING INVESTIGATED. THEIR FARTS HAVE BEEN SHOWN TO HAVE ANTIBIOTIC PROPERTIES.

RECTAL SHOUT

SMELLINESS RATING:

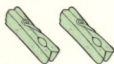

LOUDNESS RATING:

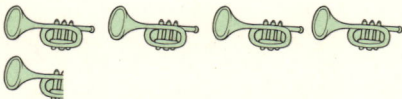

MESSINESS RATING:

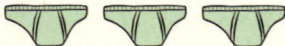

OVERALL:

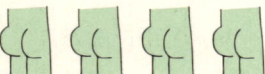

THIS IS A 12 ON THE RECTUM SCALE.
MAKE FOR COVER UNDER THE
NEAREST DOOR FRAME OR TABLE IN
THE EVENT OF AFTERSHOCKS.

MESSY FARTS

THESE ARE THE FARTS YOUR MOTHER
WARNED YOU ABOUT. NONE ARE TO BE
ATTEMPTED WHILST SITTING ON A WHITE
SOFA, OR, FOR THAT MATTER, ANY FURNITURE
YOU DON'T WANT TO THROW OUT.

BROWN FAIRY DUST

SMELLINESS RATING:

LOUDNESS RATING:

MESSINESS RATING:

OVERALL:

DON'T BE FOOLED BY THE CUTE
NAME, THIS ONE'S A POOPSTORM!
WE'RE TALKING LOCKDOWN! CONFINE
YOURSELF TO THE SMALLEST ROOM,
PUT ON YOUR RUBBER GLOVES AND BE
PREPARED TO MAKE A BIT OF A MESS.
AS FARTS GO, THIS BARELY MAKES THE
FUN-O-METER AS, UNLESS YOU'RE ROUND
YOUR PARENTS' HOUSE, YOU'RE GOING TO
HAVE TO CLEAN THIS ONE UP YOURSELF.

FART JOKES

FART TONGUE-TWISTER – TRY SAYING
THIS AS FAST AS YOU CAN:

'ONE SMART FELLOW, HE FELT SMART.
TWO SMART FELLOWS, THEY BOTH
FELT SMART. THREE SMART FELLOWS,
THEY ALL FELT SMART TOGETHER!'

GLITTER BOMB

SMELLINESS RATING:

LOUDNESS RATING:

MESSINESS RATING:

OVERALL:

THIS IS WHAT HAPPENS WHEN YOU GET
A BIT TOO COCKY AND MISJUDGE THE
FORCE IN ORDER TO EXPEL YOUR GAS –
YOU GET POO GLITTER. IT BEHAVES IN THE
SAME WAY AS NORMAL GLITTER EXCEPT
THERE'S NOTHING SPARKLY ABOUT IT.

RISKY BISCUIT

SMELLINESS RATING:

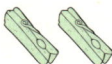

LOUDNESS RATING:

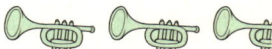

MESSINESS RATING:

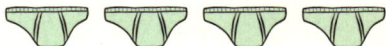

OVERALL:

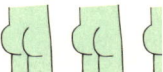

THIS FART IS NOT TO BE TRUSTED. IT'S EVEN
ODDS WHETHER A SOLID OR GAS SHOULD
BE EXPECTED, AND YOU WON'T KNOW UNTIL
IT'S MUCH, MUCH TOO LATE. THIS ONE IS FOR
DESPERADOES AND DAREDEVILS ONLY.

FARTING ETIQUETTE

FOR THE HORRORS OF A PARTICULARLY LOUD FART, YOU HAVE TO GET CREATIVE. ATTEMPT TO SHUFFLE YOUR SHOE ON THE FLOOR IN THE HOPE THAT IT TOO WILL SQUEAK. IF YOU KNOW THAT IT'S APPROACHING AND THERE'S NOTHING YOU CAN DO TO STOP IT, TRY TO MASK THE SOUND WITH A HEFTY COUGHING FIT.

POWER-SHOWER FART

SMELLINESS RATING:

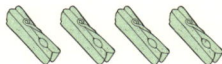

LOUDNESS RATING:

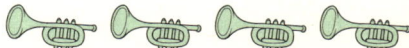

MESSINESS RATING:

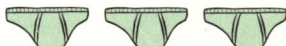

OVERALL:

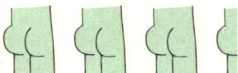

WE'VE ALL BEEN THERE – YOU'RE IN THE SHOWER, YOU'RE RELAXED AND DAYDREAMING ABOUT THE MAGICAL PLACES THE DAY MIGHT TAKE YOU. THEN, SUDDENLY, A THUNDEROUS NOISE ECHOES AROUND THE CUBICLE. FROM WHENCE? YOUR BEHIND, OF COURSE. BE SURE TO CHECK THE SURFACE BEHIND YOU DOESN'T NEED A BIT OF A RINSE OFF AFTERWARDS.

BEING CARTED OFF

SMELLINESS RATING:

LOUDNESS RATING:

MESSINESS RATING:

OVERALL:

AN UNEXPECTED FART BROUGHT ABOUT BY A HEARTY COUGH. THIS COUGH-FART HYBRID (OR 'CART') IS VERY MUCH A DOUBLE-EDGED SWORD, AS ALTHOUGH THE AUDIO CAMOUFLAGE CAN COME IN HANDY, THE COMPLETELY INVOLUNTARY NATURE OF THIS FART CAN LEAD TO IT BEING A BIT... MESSY.

DID YOU KNOW?

THE YANOMAMI TRIBE IN SOUTH
AMERICA USES FLATULENCE
AS A GREETING.

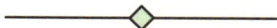

◇

TERMITE FARTS CONTRIBUTE
BETWEEN 2 AND 22 TRILLION
GRAMS OF METHANE TO THE
ATMOSPHERE EVERY YEAR.

THE SWAMP THING

SMELLINESS RATING:

LOUDNESS RATING:

MESSINESS RATING:

OVERALL:

A PERFECT TROPICAL STORM IN YOUR UNDERPANTS. THE RIGHT COMBINATION OF HUMID WEATHER, RICH, SPICY FOOD AND A SENSITIVE STOMACH LEADING TO UNSPEAKABLE REGRET IN OPTING FOR THE WHITE COTTON TROUSERS TODAY.

FART JOKES

TWO NOVICE NUNS ARE PREPARING TO BE INITIATED INTO THEIR ORDER. THEIR MOTHER SUPERIOR TELLS THEM TO GO AND COMMIT ONE SIN TO GET RID OF ANY URGES TO PERFORM UNHOLY ACTS IN THE FUTURE. THEY RETURN THE NEXT DAY, THE FIRST NUN LOOKING VERY UPSET AND THE SECOND SMILING SLYLY.

'WELL SISTERS, WHAT DID YOU DO?' ASKS THEIR MOTHER SUPERIOR.

'I ACTED IN ANGER AND SHOUTED AT AN OLD LADY ON THE BUS,' SAYS THE FIRST. 'I FELT SO BAD I SPENT ALL NIGHT CRYING INTO MY PILLOW.'

AT THIS, THE SECOND NUN'S SMILE BURSTS INTO FULL-BLOWN LAUGHTER.

'AND SISTER, WHAT DID YOU DO? WHY ARE YOU LAUGHING?' ASKS THE SENIOR NUN.

'I FARTED ON HER PILLOW!'

ADVANCED FARTING

THIS MIXED BUMBAG OF FARTS IS FULL
OF EXPULSIONS ONLY TO BE TRIED
BY TRUE EXPERTS IN FLATULENCE.

BROWN THUNDER

SMELLINESS RATING:

LOUDNESS RATING:

MESSINESS RATING:

OVERALL:

'WHOA THERE! YOU'RE GOING TO FRIGHTEN THE HORSES!' IS A CRY YOU CAN EXPECT TO HEAR WHEN YOU LET OFF ONE OF THESE DECIBEL-LADEN UNDERPANT-SCORCHERS. THE ELEMENT OF DANGER, AND THE RISK OF A BROWN STAIN, MEANS THIS IS ONE FOR PEOPLE WHO LIKE TO LIVE ON THE EDGE. VOLUME CAN BE EASILY ADJUSTED BY VARYING THE SITTING SURFACE – METAL AND WOOD BEING PARTICULARLY EXCELLENT AMPLIFIERS.

DID YOU KNOW?

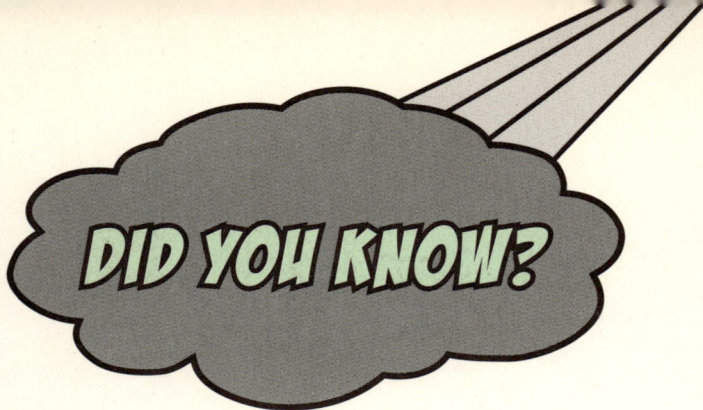

THE AVERAGE TEMPERATURE OF
A FART IS 37°C (OR 98.6°F).

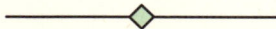

◇

THE TERM 'RASPBERRY', MEANING
TO MAKE A SOUND LIKE A FART
WITH THE MOUTH, IS AN INSTANCE
OF RHYMING SLANG, AS 'FART'
RHYMES WITH 'RASPBERRY TART'.

SNAP, CACKLE AND... PLOP

SMELLINESS RATING:

LOUDNESS RATING:

MESSINESS RATING:

OVERALL:

THIS IS THE MALODOROUS RESULT OF HOLDING IT IN FOR TOO LONG AS YOU SHUFFLE UNCOMFORTABLY ON A CHAIR, USUALLY IN ONE OF THOSE POTENTIALLY LIFE-CHANGING MOMENTS, LIKE WHEN YOU'RE MAKING YOUR DEBUT APPEARANCE ON *QUESTION TIME*. IT'S COMING AND YOU JUST CAN'T STOP IT. IT'S LIKE AN EARTHQUAKE IN YOUR PANTS, ALL YOU CAN DO IS LAUGH IT OFF AND THEN, JUST WHEN YOU THINK YOU'VE GOT AWAY WITH IT, YOU SUDDENLY FEEL TALLER AND THE CHAIR IS A BIT DAMP.

119

THE FOG

SMELLINESS RATING:

LOUDNESS RATING:

MESSINESS RATING:

OVERALL:

IF YOU LIVE WITHIN SIGHT OF A
BUSY SHIPPING LANE, YOU'LL NEED
TO HOLD THIS ONE IN UNTIL YOU
CAN DISPOSE OF IT SENSIBLY.

FART JOKES

WHAT IS A FART?

A ROYAL SALUTE, HERALDING THE
ARRIVAL OF CAPTAIN TURD.

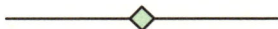

**WHAT DO YOU CALL A MAN WITH
DIARRHOEA WHO ATTEMPTS A FART?**

BRAVE.

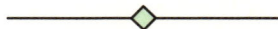

**WHAT SMELLS AND GLOWS
IN THE DARK?**

A KLINGON FART.

FREE JACUZZI

SMELLINESS RATING:

LOUDNESS RATING:

MESSINESS RATING:

OVERALL:

THERE'S NO NEED TO GO TO THE EXPENSE OF PURCHASING A TOP-OF-THE-RANGE BATHROOM SUITE WHEN YOU CAN MAKE YOUR OWN BOTTOM BUBBLES – NOW'S NOT THE TIME TO FOLLOW THROUGH UNLESS YOU WANT TO SWIM WITH POO FISH.

SCOTCH MIST

SMELLINESS RATING:

LOUDNESS RATING:

MESSINESS RATING:

OVERALL:

NO, THAT'S NOT THE DISTANT SOUND
OF BAGPIPES ECHOING ACROSS
THE HIGHLANDS – IT'S A FART WITH
THE POWER TO BLUR YOUR VISION
AND MAKE YOU SEE FAIRIES.

FARTING ETIQUETTE

FLATULENCE IN THE SWIMMING POOL: THIS CAN BE DANGEROUS IF YOU'RE IN A PUBLIC POOL THAT'S NOT SO BUSY THAT THE EXTRA BUBBLES WON'T GO UNNOTICED. IF SO, THEN TRY TO HOLD IT IN, OR AT LEAST SPLASH ABOUT A BIT AS YOU LET IT GO TO PROVIDE YOURSELF SOME COVER. IF, HOWEVER, YOU'RE IN YOUR PRIVATE HOLIDAY POOL THEN LET IT RIP.

THE LEGENDS OF FARTING

SOME FARTS NEVER DIE,
THEY LIVE ON IN INFAMY. FARTS
OF THE ORIGINALS, THE ICONS AND
THE GREATS. THESE ARE THOSE FARTS.

THE MARILYN

SMELLINESS RATING:

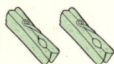

LOUDNESS RATING:

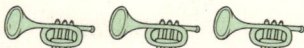

MESSINESS RATING:

OVERALL:

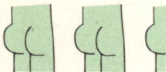

A SOPHISTICATED FART FROM A BYGONE ERA.
COMPLETELY SILENT, YET WITH THE FORCE
TO SEND A LONG DRESS FLUTTERING UP
AROUND YOUR EARS. YOU DIDN'T THINK THAT
WAS WIND FROM AN AIR VENT, DID YOU?

THE ELVIS

SMELLINESS RATING:

LOUDNESS RATING:

MESSINESS RATING:

OVERALL:

A FART GUARANTEED TO GET SCORES OF
TEENAGE GIRLS SCREAMING AND PASSING
OUT. GET YOUR HIPS SHAKING AND LIP
SNARLING AND LET OUT A FART THAT'LL
LEAVE YOU ALL SHOOK UP. IF YOU'RE
MET WITH ANY DISAPPROVING GLANCES,
JUST BLAME IT ON THE HOUND DOG.

DID YOU KNOW?

ONE OF THE CLASSIC FARTS IN LITERATURE APPEARS IN GEOFFREY CHAUCER'S *THE CANTERBURY TALES*, WRITTEN IN THE LATE FOURTEENTH CENTURY. A CHARACTER NAMED NICHOLAS BREAKS WIND IN THE FACE OF ABSALOM, A PARISH CLERK, BEFORE ABSALOM BRANDS NICHOLAS ON THE BUTTOCKS.

THE JAGGER

SMELLINESS RATING:

LOUDNESS RATING:

MESSINESS RATING:

OVERALL:

WEARING SKIN-TIGHT PANTS
AND STRUTTING IN SIX-INCH HEELS
IS NOT GOING TO STOP ONE OF
THESE FROM ROCKING OUT
OF YOUR ANAL PASSAGE – IT'S A
GAS, GAS, GAAAAAAASSSS!

ANIMAL FARTS

IF A BEAR FARTS IN THE FOREST, DOES HE LAUGH? NO. AND THAT'S WHAT SEPARATES US FROM THE ANIMALS. THESE FARTS ALL HELP TO BRIDGE THE GAP BETWEEN MAN AND BEAST.

CHIPMUNK

SMELLINESS RATING:

LOUDNESS RATING:

MESSINESS RATING:

OVERALL:

THIS ONE HAS QUITE A GUTTURAL SOUND, THE WAY IT STOPS AND STARTS AND YOU'RE NEVER SURE IF YOU'VE FINISHED. IT'S LIKE YOUR BEHIND IS CHEWING A TOFFEE.

FART JOKES

TWO OLD MEN ARE IN A CAFE EATING LUNCH. ONE OLD MAN, WHO HAS JUST MOVED IN WITH HIS SON AND DAUGHTER-IN-LAW, IS TELLING THE OTHER ABOUT ALL THE GREAT TECHNOLOGY IN HIS NEW HOME.

'WHEN I GET UP IN THE NIGHT TO GO TO THE BATHROOM, THE LIGHT TURNS ON BY ITSELF!'

INTRIGUED BY THIS, THE OTHER OLD MAN WAITS FOR HIS FRIEND'S FAMILY TO PICK HIM UP AND ASKS ABOUT THIS BRILLIANT INNOVATION. THE FRIEND'S SON, WITH A LOOK OF REALISATION ON HIS FACE, EXCLAIMS, 'SO HE'S THE ONE WHO'S BEEN MAKING A MESS IN THE FRIDGE!'

BUFFALO

SMELLINESS RATING:

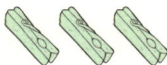

LOUDNESS RATING:

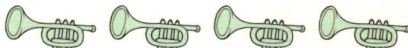

MESSINESS RATING:

OVERALL:

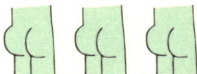

A BIG, BEEFY, WOOLLY FART – THE PERFECT
TRUMP EMPLOYED BY MANY AN AFTER-
DINNER SPEAKER TO SOUND THE END OF A
ROUSING SPEECH, WORTHY OF A STANDING
OVATION IN ANYBODY'S LANGUAGE.

HYENA

SMELLINESS RATING:

LOUDNESS RATING:

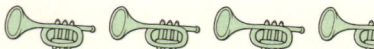

MESSINESS RATING:

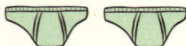

OVERALL:

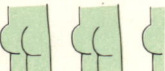

THIS FART SOUNDS LIKE YOUR ANUS
IS LAUGHING AT YOU, AS IF MOCKING
YOU FOR TRYING TO HOLD IT IN. IT'S
A WILD ONE, THAT'S FOR SURE.

THE AMOUNT WE FART CAN BE
INCREASED BY DRINKING FIZZY
DRINKS AND CHEWING GUM. THIS IS
BECAUSE THESE TWO ACTIVITIES
INCREASE THE AMOUNT OF GAS
IN OUR DIGESTIVE SYSTEM BY
INGESTING THE CARBONATION IN
THE DRINKS AND SWALLOWING
AIR WHILST CHEWING THE GUM.

THE WHALE SONG

SMELLINESS RATING:

LOUDNESS RATING:

MESSINESS RATING:

OVERALL:

A FART MUCH LIKE ITS NAMESAKE –
MAJESTIC, MYSTERIOUS AND UNHURRIED.
A LONG, DEEP, SONOROUS FART THAT
WILL CARRY FOR MILES AROUND. BE
CAREFUL LETTING THIS ONE GO IN
THE BATH AS YOU MAY END UP IN AN
AWKWARD CONVERSATION WITH A GIANT
MARINE MAMMAL YOU'VE NEVER MET.

THE PARROT

SMELLINESS RATING:

LOUDNESS RATING:

MESSINESS RATING:

OVERALL:

A FART ONLY TO BE ATTEMPTED BY
TRUE MASTERS OF THE FLATUS. WITH
THIS EXPULSION, THE FARTER TRIES TO
IMITATE OTHER SOUNDS, LIKE THE UNHOLY
COMBINATION OF LE PÉTOMANE (WELL-
KNOWN FRENCH TURN-OF-THE-CENTURY
FLATULIST, OR FART ENTERTAINER)
AND THAT GUY FROM *POLICE ACADEMY*
WHO DID THE SOUND EFFECTS.

FART JOKES

AT A DINNER PARTY, A MAN FEELS THE NEED TO FART AND JUST CAN'T HOLD IT IN. THINKING HE GOT AWAY WITH IT, HE RELAXES SLIGHTLY UNTIL THE WOMAN SITTING NEXT TO HIM EXCLAIMS, 'I CAN'T BELIEVE YOU FARTED IN FRONT OF ME!'

TO WHICH THE MAN REPLIES, 'I'M SORRY, I DIDN'T THINK IT WAS YOUR TURN.'

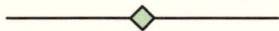

◆

WHICH SERIAL KILLER FARTED THE MOST?

JACK THE RIPPER.

THE VAMPIRE BAT

SMELLINESS RATING:

LOUDNESS RATING:

MESSINESS RATING:

OVERALL:

A FART SHROUDED IN MYSTERY AND SUPERSTITION. GENERALLY NOCTURNAL, THIS FART ELICITS A STRONG RESPONSE FROM ANYONE WHO GETS A WHIFF. ITS STINK IS SUCH THAT THE BLOOD WILL DRAIN COMPLETELY FROM THEIR FACES, LEAVING THEM PALE AND SICKLY. LEGEND HAS IT THAT IF YOU'RE 'BITTEN' BY THE VAMPIRE BAT, YOU'VE ONLY HOURS LEFT BEFORE YOU TURN, AND FART ONE YOURSELF...

THE RATTLE SNAKE

SMELLINESS RATING:

LOUDNESS RATING:

MESSINESS RATING:

OVERALL:

A VENOMOUS FART, CAPABLE OF CAUSING UNTOLD DAMAGE TO ANYONE SUBJECTED TO IT. THE KEY WARNING SIGNS THAT YOU'RE ABOUT TO UNLEASH A RATTLER ARE A RATTLE-LIKE GURGLE EMANATING FROM YOUR DIGESTIVE SYSTEM, FOLLOWED BY A HISS AS IT IS SLOWLY RELEASED. BY THE TIME IT'S BEEN SMELT, IT'S MUCH TOO LATE; PARALYSIS HAS SET IN AND DEATH IS INEVITABLE.

THE NIGHT OWL

SMELLINESS RATING:

LOUDNESS RATING:

MESSINESS RATING:

OVERALL:

THIS ONE IS A NIGHT-TIME TOOT THAT'LL CHILL YOU TO THE BONE. PUNGENT ENOUGH TO MAKE YOU TURN YOUR HEAD ALL THE WAY AROUND AND LEAVE YOU WIDE-EYED AND WIDE AWAKE, WONDERING WHETHER THAT NOISE WAS A SPOOKY VISITOR OUTSIDE YOUR WINDOW OR A STINKY VISITOR INSIDE YOUR PANTS.

THE FINAL FART

THE LONG FART GOODNIGHT

SMELLINESS RATING:

LOUDNESS RATING:

MESSINESS RATING:

OVERALL:

FOR WHEN A KISS
ISN'T NEARLY ENOUGH...
SURE TO LEAVE A
LASTING IMPRESSION!

IF YOU'RE INTERESTED IN FINDING
OUT MORE ABOUT OUR BOOKS,
FIND US ON FACEBOOK AT
SUMMERSDALE PUBLISHERS
AND FOLLOW US ON TWITTER AT
@SUMMERSDALE.

WWW.SUMMERSDALE.COM